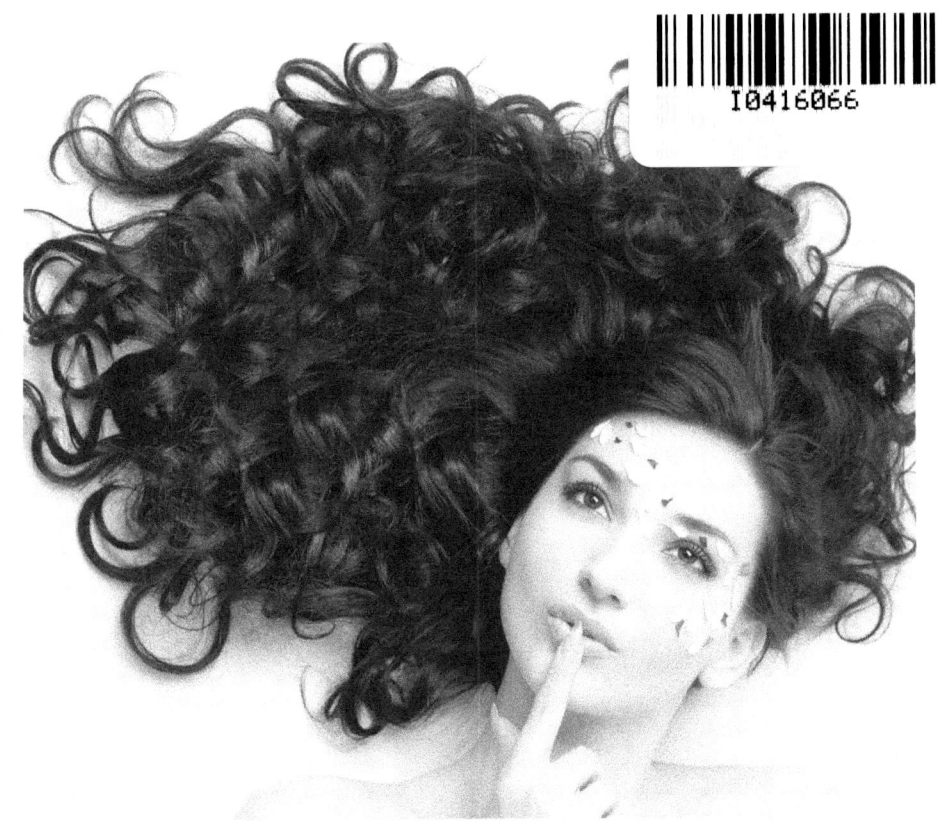

Secret

Hair Growth

Recipes

Secret Beauty Recipes Volume 2 concentrates on hair growth & strengthening oils, serum, masks & moisture treatments. These historic recipes were hand-picked just for you. The treatments are easy to blend together, safe, economical and beneficial for dryness, flakes, scalp restoration & to promote faster hair growth. Bonus recipes are included for a whole body experience.

Contents

Basic ingredient Information

ALWAYS try a small amount of product on your wrist 24 hours before using to make sure you're not allergic to the ingredients.

When making cosmetics use a porcelain or glass pot, because stainless steel cooking pots can potentially leach poisonous heavy metals into your mixtures. Nonmetal is best for working with herbs and oils.

- Strawberries are a great ingredient to use in face masks, since they're packed with vitamin C. They are also rich in alpha-hydroxy acids that help exfoliate the skin. So fresh strawberry masks are great for people with dull, damaged or acne-prone skin.

- Honey is a natural humectant, helping to hold moisture in the skin; it also has antibacterial, antifungal, antiviral & antioxidant properties.

- Almond oil is a natural, skin-softening emollient that is easily absorbed by the skin.

- Cucumber adds vitamins A and C and antioxidants.

- Carrots can tone and clarify your skin, since they are naturally antiseptic and packed with vitamins (like carotene) and iron.

- Aloe helps stimulate new hair growth, fights frizz and works as a natural conditioner.

- Birch can help combat dry, itchy scalp.

- Burdock helps promotes hair growth, increases shine, body & fights dandruff.

- Chamomile works really well as a natural conditioner. It can also lighten blonde hair over time.

- Licorice traditionally been associated with preventing hair loss.

- Marigold acts as wonderful moisturizer. It can help lighten your natural hair color & increase shine.

- Mulberries have historically been used to treat premature gray hair.

- Pomegranate seed oil revitalizes dull strands and increases flexibility.

- Parsley is full of iron & vitamin C which help keep hair healthy and strong.

- Sage can works as a natural coloring agent & also fight gray hair.

- Rice bran contains vitamin E which creates a type of shell around the cuticle so your strands have less breakage.

- Hemp seed oil is packed with amino acids, omega-3 fatty acids, proteins, and minerals that make hair stronger and healthier overall.

- Bananas are high in Vitamin C, A, B6 and B12, plus they contain potassium and magnesium. The fruit acids in bananas help slough off dead skin and energize the complexion.

- Avocado oil is excellent for the hair because it is rich in proteins and amino acids, and it has high levels of vitamins A, D, and E, The proteins help fill in all the crevices in your hair's cuticles, so each strand is stronger and better protected from future breakage.

- Coconut oil is historically known to be one of the best moisture-retaining hair conditioners on earth. Coconut oil can cleanse, moisturizes and stimulate the growth of hair follicles

- Sweet Potatoes have amazing anti-aging, anti-wrinkling benefits.

-

- It is rich in fiber, beta-carotene (vitamin A equivalent which fights free radicals in the body) and vitamin C, iron apart from vitamin B6, magnesium, phosphorus, potassium, sodium and zinc.

- Sweet almond has high contents of vitamins A, B, and E. It helps heal split ends, improves circulation in the scalp to produce stronger hair, and can add luster and shine to dull hair: "The fatty acids also add UV protection by reflecting harmful rays.

- Rosemary oil is great for mixing with other oils because it stimulates the hair follicles It is also, high in iron, calcium, and vitamin B, the oil acts as an anti-aging agent, which helps boost color, shine, thickness, and prevents hair loss.

- Almond oil is a rich source of Vitamin-E and hence you will see it in a lot of my recipes. Regular massaging promotes strong, long, shiny and thick hair and happy scalp.

- Olive oil possesses anti-fungal and anti-bacterial properties which aid in destroying bacteria in your scalp thereby promoting hair growth. It helps to restore scalp cell health, nourish, condition & improve elasticity and strength.

Restorative Hair Serum

- 1 T Olive Oil
- 5 drops Sage oil
- 5 drops ylang-ylang oil
- 5 drops tea tree oil
- 5 drops Bay oil
- 5 drops Lavender oil

Mix all oils in a dark bottle. Store finished product in the refrigerator. Use daily for scalp moisture. Use also as a deep penetrating oil treatment under hot cap, steamer or dryer for 20 minutes.

Stimulating Shine Hair Serum

- 4 Once Jojoba Oil
- 5 drops Sage oil
- 5 drops Rosemary oil
- 5 drops Peppermint oil
- 5 drops Tea Tree oil

Mix oils in a bottle & store in cool dark place. Use daily for scalp moisture. Use also as a deep penetrating oil treatment under hot cap, steamer or dryer.

Apple Vinegar Growth Rinse

- 1 T Apple Vinegar
- 1 t mustard seed oil
- 16 oz. of water

Mix ingredients well. Pour over hair massage into scalp. Rinse hair weekly to promote growth.

Garlic Hair Growth Recipe

Aloe is a wonderful natural hair product because it helps repair & restore damaged hair. It is also a natural astringent, which helps remove excess dirt and oil, too.
It is very moisturizing & soothing if you suffer from dandruff or dry skin.

- 5 cups water
- 1 chamomile tea bag
- 1 peppermint tea bag
- 1 T garlic juice
- 1 t olive oil
- 1 T honey
- 1 T aloe gel
- 1 egg yolk

Steep the tea bags for 5 minutes. Blend half the tea with other ingredients until smooth. Massage the mixture into hair & scalp for 5 minutes. Apply plastic and dryer, warm towel or steamer for 20 minutes. Rinse once then do a final rinse of the hair with the other half of the tea. Rinse well and no-poo as usual.

Jojoba/ Honey Hair Growth Oil

Need extra moisture on a daily basis? Here it is! Jojoba oil has the ability to condition hair, repair its texture & shine. Lavender oil, like aloe soothes irritated scalps and encourages hair growth.

- 1 T jojoba oil
- 1 T honey
- 1 T aloe gel
- 3 drops lavender oil
- 1 t olive oil
- 3 drops tea tree oil
- 3 drops sage
- 3 drops lavender
- 3 drops rosemary

Blend all ingredients well. Pour in small bottle. Apply to scalp nightly and massage 5 minutes.

Vitamin E Hair Growth Recipe

- 1/4 cup of vitamin E oil
- 1/4 cup of jojoba oil
- 2 drops mustard seed oil
- 6 drops of rosemary essential oil
- 10 drops of peppermint essential oil
- 1 T vitamin E oil
- 1 T olive oil
- 1 t aloe oil

Blend all ingredients well. Pour in small bottle. Apply to scalp and massage 5 minutes. .

Daily Wild Growth Oil

These oils have been historically used on the scalps of men, women & children for generations to avoid dryness, flaking and breakage.

- 2 drop mustard seed oil
- 1 T vitamin e
- 2 drops thyme essential oil
- 2 drops lavender essential oil
- 2 drops tea tree oil
- 2 drops rosemary essential oil
- 2 drops cedar essential oil
- 1/2 oz. grape seed oil
- 1 t jojoba oil

Blend all ingredients until mixed well. Store in an airtight container and massage into the scalp twice a day.

Simple Honey Hair moisture Mask

Try this treatment for 1 hour, once a week for a month.

- 1 T olive oil
- 1/2 cup of honey

Mix well. Add to your fresh-washed hair. Wait for twenty minutes and then rinse thoroughly with warm water.

Simple Honey Hair Moisture Mist

- 1 t honey
- 1 t Olive oil
- 1 cup water

Blend well. Pour into spray bottle to use as a leave-in conditioner.

Nettle Rosemary Root Stimulator

- 1/2 oz. nettle
- 1/2 oz. peppermint
- 2 cups of water
- 1T rosemary
- 2 cups of white wine vinegar
- 1T mustard seed oil

Simmer nettle, rosemary & peppermint for two hours. Cool and strain. Stir in the oils and pour into a bottle. Shake well before every use. Massage into your scalp every other night.

Olive Oil Honey Super Moisture Treatment

- 1 T Kukui butter
- 1 T vitamin E
- 2 T olive oil
- 3 T honey
- 1/2 cup coconut milk
- 1/2 avocado
- 1 egg yolk

Blend all ingredients until smooth. Apply to dry hair for 20 minutes with steam or warm towel. Rinse well.

Honey Hair Strength Treatment

This deep conditioning mask can help revitalize your hair & scalp plus protect your hair from damage & breaking.

- 1 T honey
- 1 t mustard seed oil
- 1 t cinnamon
- 1 T olive oil
- 1 T Almond oil

Mix well. Apply to your hair root to tip. Massage into scalp for 5 minutes, then wait 15 minutes and rinse.

Apple Cider Vinegar Conditioner

Vinegar helps soften hair and makes it shine. The apple cider vinegar scent will fade away completely when your hair dries.

- 4 eggs
- 2 T grape seed oil
- 2 T vegetable glycerin
- 1 cup water
- 2 t apple cider vinegar

Whip all ingredients in a blender until smooth. Massage into freshly shampooed hair and scalp. Leave on for up to 15 minutes, and then rinse thoroughly.

Deep-Conditioning Honey & Yogurt Hair Mask

All of the ingredients in this recipe moisturize and soften your hair.

- 2 eggs, beaten
- 1 cup plain yogurt
- 2 T grape seed oil (or olive oil)
- 1 T honey

Whip all ingredients in a blender until smooth. Apply to dry hair, concentrating on hair ends. Wait for 15-20 minutes,

Hydrating Avocado Hair Mask

- 1 banana
- 1 egg yolk
- 1 t maple syrup
- 1/2 avocado
- 1 t olive oil
- 1 t Shea butter

Blend ingredients until smooth. Apply and let dry 30-45 minutes. Shower off. .

Horsetail Strengthening Mask

The horsetail herb is a great source of silica. Silica will strengthen your hair at its core and help restore shine.

- 2 T horsetail
- 1 t olive oil
- 1 t aloe
- ½ banana
- 1 avocado

Steep horsetail in 1 cup of water for 5 minutes, blend other ingredients until smooth. Apply to hair, root to tip. Let dry. Rinse out with warm water. Shampoo or no-poo your hair as usual.

Onion Scalp Mask

Onion has the benefits of the high sulfur content. Mustard seed oil has traditionally been used to stimulate the hair follicle.
This mixture can help stimulate hair growth!

- 1/4 cup Onion juice
- 6 t Olive oil
- 3 t Vitamin E
- 1 t mustard seed oil

Just blend some onions in your food processor and extract the juice; Mix with other ingredients until smooth.
Apply this on your scalp and leave for at least 30 minutes or more.
Rinse with warm water and shampoo or no-poo as usual

Sweet potato hair mask

- 1 sweet potato
- 3 T Olive oil
- 1 Cup of yogurt
- 2 T honey

Prick holes in the sweet potato with a fork and microwave for 10-12 minutes.
Alternatively, you can use Glory canned sweet potato. Combine all ingredients. Apply to hair for 20 - 30 minutes and rinse with warm water. Shampoo or no-poo as usual.

Apple/Orange/Olive oil Hair Mask

- 1 cup (1 or 2) apples
- 2 T Apple cider vinegar
- 1 t lemon juice
- 1 t orange juice
- 1 T tea tree oil
- 1 T Vitamin E
- 1 T corn flour

Peel, core and grate 1-2 large apples or use canned apples
Combine all ingredients; mix well.
Apply to dry, unwashed hair
Wait for 20-30 minutes rinse and shampoo or no-poo as usual.

Vitamin E & Almond Oil Hair Smoothing Mask

¼ cup of honey
½ cup of yogurt
1 t Olive oil
1 t Vitamin E
1 T Almond oil

Combine all ingredients, work it into your hair from root to tip. Wrap hair in plastic & leave it on for 20-30 minutes then shampoo as normal.

Egg/Olive oil Mask

- 1 T almond oil
- 1 egg yolk
- 2 T of olive oil
- 4 oz. of liquid honey
- 1 T mayonnaise

Mix the ingredients together with a stick-blender and then apply to clean, damp, towel dry hair. Apply warm towel. steamer or plastic cap for 20 minutes then rinse out with warm water.

Banana/Coconut/Honey Hair Mask

- 1 ripe Banana
- 1 T Honey
- 1 T Olive Oil
- 1/2 t Almond oil
- 1/2 t Jojoba oil
- 1 T Yogurt
- 2 T Coconut Milk
- 1 egg white
- 1 T Vitamin E butter

Combine all ingredients, work it into your hair from root to tip. Wrap hair in plastic & leave it on for 20-30 minutes then shampoo as normal.

Bonus Recipes

Organic Coconut Oil/ Raw Honey Mask

- 1 T Organic Coconut Oil
- 1 T Organic Raw Honey
- 1 t Olive Oil

Apply to dry or wet hair generously from top to bottom, focusing on the ends where most damage occurs. Wrap your hair in a warm, damp towel and let the mask soak in for 30-40 minutes. Shampoo the mask out in the shower then shampoo or no-poo and condition as normal.

Olive/Honey Dry Hair Mask

Apply this mask whenever your hair gets dry, such as in the winter & summer or after coloring & chemical services.

- 3 tbs. olive oil
- 1/2 cup honey
- 1/2 banana
- 3 T Coconut milk

Mix olive oil, milk, banana and honey. Apply to hair. Wrap your hair in a warm, damp towel. Leave the mask on for 20-30 minutes. Shampoo and rinse well.

Cucumber Hair Smoother

If you swim in a chlorinated pool for exercise on a regular basis, the same damage you've noticed happening to your skin and bathing suit, is happening to your hair, as well. Try this treatment at home to keep chlorine damage to a minimum.

- 1 T tea tree oil
- 1 egg
- 2 T olive oil
- ¼ peeled cucumber

Blend the egg, olive oil, tea tree oil & peeled cucumber.

Spread evenly through your hair, leave on for 10 minutes, then rinse.

Natural Dandruff Remedy

- 2 T of olive oil
- juice of 1/2 lemon
- juice of 1/2 lime
- 2 T of water
- 1-2 drops of Tea Tree essential oil

Mix together and massage into your damp scalp, then leave for 20 minutes before rinsing off with warm water and applying shampoo. Treat weekly.

Collard Green/Sweet Potato Soak

Collard Greens can help to prevent acne because they are rich in vitamin A which acts like a topical prescription to help exfoliate your skin naturally.

- 1/2 Cup Collard Greens
- 1/2 Sweet Potato

Add chopped greens & Sweet potato to mesh bag or foot of panty hose

(tie knot). Drop into bath and soak 20 minutes

Anti-Aging Face Mask

Sweet potatoes have some of the best anti-inflammatory properties.

Mangoes and honey fight off free radical damage that the sun causes which can cause wrinkles in our skin and premature aging.

- 1 small sweet potato
- 1 mango
- 1 T Olive oil
- 5 TB honey

Prick holes in the sweet potato with a fork and microwave for 10-12 minutes. Alternatively, you can use Glory canned sweet potato.

Scoop out mango & sweet potato and mash up. Mix all ingredients together. Once cooled, apply to whole or body. Wait for 15-20 minutes.

Shower off with warm water.

Sweet Potato Foot Soak

- 1 Sweet potato or 1 can of Glory brand
- 6 drops of tea tree oil
- 3 T Olive oil
- 3 t Almond oil

Prick holes in the sweet potato with a fork and microwave for 10-12 minutes.

Alternatively, you can use canned sweet potato. Boil sweet potatoes. Let water cool, Add tea tree, almond oil & olive oil soak feet in the water 10-15 minutes. It will soften your heels like nothing else.

Sweet potato/Olive oil/Nutmeg Mask

- 2 ounces of mashed sweet potatoes (or 1 can of Glory)
- 1 tablespoons of oatmeal
- 1 tablespoon of honey
- 1 T Olive oil
- A dash of nutmeg

Mix ingredients all together to form a thick paste.

Apply the mixture onto clean face, neck, and chest.

Let it sit for 5-10 minutes before showering off with warm water

Sweet Potato Body Mask

- 1 sweet potato
- 1 T virgin coconut oil (or olive oil)
- 1 t sour cream (or plain yogurt)
- 3 T raw honey

Prick holes in the sweet potato with a fork and microwave for 10-12 minutes.

Alternatively, you can use Glory canned sweet potato. Place in a food processor or blender. Add coconut oil, sour cream and honey then, blend until you have an extremely smooth texture. Apply all over the body & wait for 20 minutes.

Shower off. Apply your favorite toner and moisturizer to lock in softness.

Avocado Cream Mask

This mask will rebuild skin collagen, improve tone and texture, and fade age spots.

- 1 t olive oil
- 1 avocado, mashed
- 1 carrot, cooked and mashed
- 1/2 cup heavy cream
- 1 egg, beaten
- 2 tablespoons honey

Combine all ingredients in a bowl until smooth. Spread gently over your face, hair and neck, and leave in place 10-15 minutes. Rinse with cool water and follow with your favorite toner.

Kukui/Neem Daily Scalp Butter

- 1/4 ounce kukui butter
- 1/4 ounce neem butter
- 1/8 ounce jojoba oil
- 1/4 ounce vitamin e
- 1/4 ounce broccoli seed oil
- 1/4 ounce carrot oil
- 1/4 ounce watermelon seed oil

Melt butters & Combine all ingredients in a measuring cup and mix well.

Quick Strawberry Moisturizing Mask

- 8 - 9 Fresh strawberries
- 2 T of honey
- 1 t Extra virgin olive,
- 1 t grape seed
- 1 t sweet almond oil
- Few drops of fresh lemon juice - About 4 drops if you have dry skin and up to 1 tablespoon for oily skin.

Mix honey, oils, and lemon juice until well-incorporated. Gently apply over your body, avoiding the eye area. Relax and leave the mask on for 5 minutes. Gently wash it away with warm face cloth & water, pat your face dry.

Apple moisture mask

- 1 T Olive oil
- 1 t heavy Cream
- 1 T Wheat Germ
- 1/2 red apple

Purée apple w/ olive oil & cream in a blender or add applesauce to a small bowl.

Mix in the wheat germ to form a paste.

Apply to clean face. Allow mask to set for 10-15 minutes

Banana and Milk Face Mask

- 1/2 banana, mashed
- 1 T honey
- 1 t Olive oil
- 1 T whole milk
- 1 t heavy cream

Mix all ingredients until smooth and creamy.

Apply to face for 15 minutes & rinse with warm water.

Green tea/goat milk/salt bath

- 3 teabags
- 3 T Coconut Milk
- 3 tablespoons of dry goat milk
- 3 tablespoons of course salt (kosher or sea salt)

Mix all ingredients until smooth and creamy.

This is my Favorite! It leaves the body super soft and relaxed